CANCER PREVENTION AND EARLY DETECTION

The Importance of Regular check-ups
and Healthy Habits

Diane T. Norwood

Copyright © 2023 Diane T. Norwood

All rights reserved.

ISBN: 9798376490525

DEDICATION

"To those who have lost loved ones to cancer, and to those who are fighting it every day. May this book empower you with knowledge and hope, and may it inspire us all to take action towards a future free of this disease."

CONTENTS

CANCER

Cancer is a disease characterized by the uncontrolled growth of cells in the body. It can develop in any part of the body and can spread to other areas if left untreated. There are many different types of cancer, each with its own unique symptoms, causes, and treatments. One of the biggest challenges with cancer is that it can take years, or even decades, for the disease to develop and become symptomatic. This makes early detection and treatment crucial for the best outcomes. The good news is that there are many things that individuals can do to reduce their risk of developing cancer, including making healthy lifestyle choices, getting regular preventive screenings, and seeking medical attention for any potential symptoms. A healthy diet and regular physical activity have been shown to reduce the risk of many types of cancer. Eating a diet rich in fruits, vegetables, and whole grains, and avoiding processed foods, red meat, and excessive alcohol consumption can help reduce the risk of developing cancer. Regular physical activity, such as walking or cycling, can also lower the risk. In addition to making healthy lifestyle choices, regular preventive screenings can help catch cancer early, when it is most treatable. These can include mammograms, colonoscopies, and pap smears, as well as tests for other types of cancer, such as prostate cancer or skin

"

cancer. It is important to understand your personal risk factors and talk to your doctor about the right screenings for you. It is also important to be aware of any potential symptoms of cancer and seek medical attention if needed. Some common symptoms include changes in bowel or bladder habits, unusual bleeding or discharge, persistent pain, and changes in skin, nails, or moles. Family history and genetics also play a role in cancer risk. If you have a family history of cancer, it is important to talk to your doctor about your personal risk and any preventive measures that may be necessary. Additionally, the HPV vaccine has been shown to reduce the risk of certain types of cancer, including cervical cancer. Finally, it is important to stay informed and up-to-date on the latest cancer research and advances in treatment. This can include attending educational events, reading reliable sources, and talking to your doctor about your options. With the right resources and support, individuals can take steps to prevent cancer and catch it early, when it is most treatable. Cancer is a complex and serious disease that can have a profound impact on individuals and their families. However, there are many things that individuals can do to reduce their risk of developing cancer and improve their outcomes. By making healthy lifestyle choices, getting regular preventive screenings, and seeking medical attention for any potential symptoms, individuals can take control of their health and reduce the impact of cancer.

IMPORTANCE OF REGULAR CANCER SCREENINGS

Cancer is a disease that affects millions of people around the world. It is a complex disease that can have a profound impact on individuals and their families, and it can be challenging to treat, especially if it is not detected early. This is why cancer prevention and early detection are so important. Preventing cancer starts with making healthy lifestyle choices. A healthy diet that is rich in fruits, vegetables, and whole grains, and low in processed foods, red meat, and alcohol, can help reduce the risk of developing cancer. Regular physical activity, such as walking or cycling, can also help lower the risk. Additionally, avoiding tobacco and excessive alcohol consumption are important steps in reducing the risk of cancer. Another important aspect of cancer prevention is getting regular preventive screenings. Screenings, such as mammograms, colonoscopies, and pap smears, can help detect cancer early when it is most treatable. It is important to understand your personal risk factors and talk to your doctor about the right screenings for you. For example, if you have a family history of colon cancer, your doctor may recommend more frequent colonoscopies. Early detection is also crucial for improving outcomes in the treatment of cancer. When cancer is detected early, it is typically smaller and has not yet spread to other parts of the body. This means that the treatment options are often more effective and less invasive, and the chances of a positive outcome are much higher. In addition to regular preventive screenings, it is also important to be aware of any potential symptoms of cancer and seek medical attention if needed. Some common symptoms include changes in bowel or bladder habits, unusual bleeding or discharge, persistent pain, and changes in skin, nails, or moles. If you are experiencing any of these symptoms, it is important to talk to your doctor to rule out cancer and get the appropriate treatment if needed. Family history and genetics also play a role in cancer risk. If you have a family history of cancer, it is important to talk to your doctor about your personal risk and any preventive measures that may be necessary. Additionally, the HPV vaccine has been shown to reduce the risk of certain types of cancer, including cervical cancer. It is also important to stay informed and up-to-date on the latest cancer research and advances in treatment. This can include attending educational events, reading reliable sources, and talking to your doctor about your options. With the right resources and support, individuals can take steps to prevent cancer and catch it early, when it is most treatable. Finally, cancer prevention and early detection are important not only for the individual but also for society as a whole. Early detection and effective treatment can reduce the financial burden of cancer treatment on individuals and the healthcare system, as well as improve the overall quality of life for those affected by the disease. Cancer prevention and early detection are crucial for reducing the impact of this disease. By making healthy lifestyle choices, getting regular preventive screenings, and seeking medical attention for any potential symptoms, individuals can take control of their health and improve their chances of a positive outcome. Additionally, staying informed and up-to-date on the latest cancer research and advances in treatment can help individuals make the best decisions for their health and well-being.

ROLE OF HEALTHY LIFESTYLE CHOICES (E.G. DIET, EXERCISE, AVOIDING TOBACCO)

A healthy lifestyle is crucial for reducing the risk of developing cancer and improving overall health. By making healthy choices, such as following a nutritious diet, engaging in regular physical activity, and avoiding tobacco, individuals can greatly impact their health and well-being. Starting with diet, eating a diet rich in fruits, vegetables, and whole grains can help reduce the risk of cancer. Fruits and vegetables contain important vitamins and minerals that support the body's immune system, and whole grains provide the fiber that can help keep the digestive system healthy. On the other hand, a diet high in processed foods, red meat, and alcohol can increase the risk of cancer. Limiting these foods and instead opting for a diet rich in whole, nutrient-dense foods can help reduce the risk of developing cancer. Physical activity is also important for cancer prevention. Engaging in regular physical activity, such as walking or cycling, can help lower the risk of cancer by supporting the body's immune system and reducing inflammation. In addition, regular physical activity can help maintain a healthy weight, which is another important factor in reducing the risk of cancer. It is recommended that individuals get at least 150 minutes of moderate-intensity physical activity per week, or 30 minutes a day, five days a week. Avoiding tobacco is also critical for reducing the risk of cancer. Tobacco use is the leading cause of preventable death worldwide and is a major risk factor for multiple types of cancer, including lung, mouth, throat, bladder, and pancreatic cancer. Quitting tobacco can significantly reduce the risk of cancer and improve overall health. Additionally, avoiding exposure to secondhand smoke can also help reduce the risk of cancer. It is important to note that making healthy lifestyle choices is not only beneficial for reducing the risk of cancer, but it also supports overall health and well-being. A healthy diet and regular physical activity can help improve mood and energy levels and reduce the risk of chronic diseases such as heart disease, stroke, and diabetes. Healthy lifestyle choices is a crucial aspect of cancer prevention. By following a nutritious diet, engaging in regular physical activity, and avoiding tobacco, individuals can greatly impact their health and well-being, and reduce the risk of developing cancer. It is never too late to make positive changes, and by making small, achievable changes, individuals can create a healthier future for themselves and their loved ones.

UNDERSTANDING FAMILY HISTORY AND GENETIC RISK FOR CANCER

Understanding family history and genetic risk for cancer is an important aspect of cancer prevention and early detection. Family history can provide valuable information about the risk of developing certain types of cancer, and genetic testing can help determine whether an individual has a genetic mutation that increases their risk of developing certain types of cancer. A family history of cancer refers to the presence of cancer in a person's blood relatives, such as parents, siblings, grandparents, or children. The risk of developing cancer can be increased if multiple family members have been diagnosed with the same or related types of cancer, particularly if the cancers occurred at a young age. For example, if several family members have been diagnosed with breast cancer, the risk of developing breast cancer may be higher in other family members. It is important to talk to family members about their medical history and share this information with healthcare providers. This information can help healthcare providers determine whether an individual is at increased risk for developing certain types of cancer and whether additional screening tests or preventive measures are needed. In some cases, a family history of cancer can be due to an inherited genetic mutation. Inherited genetic mutations are changes in DNA that are passed down from one generation to the next. These mutations can increase the risk of developing certain types of cancer, such as breast, ovarian, and colon cancer. Genetic testing can help determine whether an individual has an inherited genetic mutation that increases their risk of developing certain types of cancer. Genetic testing is typically recommended for individuals with a family history of cancer or who have other risk factors, such as a personal history of cancer at a young age. There are several types of genetic tests available, including predictive genetic testing, which is used to determine whether an individual has an increased risk of developing cancer-based on their family history, and diagnostic genetic testing, which is used to confirm a diagnosis of cancer. Genetic testing can be done through a blood test or a saliva test. It is important to consider the potential emotional impact of genetic testing and to understand the limitations of the results. For example, a positive test result does not guarantee that an individual will develop cancer, and a negative test result does not mean that the individual will not develop cancer. It is also important to consider the privacy and confidentiality of genetic test results, as well as the potential for discrimination based on genetic information. Family history and genetic risk for cancer is an important aspect of cancer prevention and early detection. Talking to family members about their medical history, undergoing genetic testing, and discussing the results with healthcare providers can help individuals determine their risk of developing certain types of cancer and make informed decisions about their health. It is important to consider the emotional impact and potential limitations of genetic testing and to take steps to protect the privacy and confidentiality of genetic information.

Importance of HPV vaccination for cancer prevention

Human Papillomavirus (HPV) is a group of viruses that can cause a range of health problems, including genital warts and various types of cancer. In particular, HPV is responsible for nearly all cases of cervical cancer and a significant proportion of anal, vaginal, penile, and oropharyngeal cancers. The HPV vaccine has been shown to be effective in preventing HPV infections and reducing the risk of HPV-related cancers. The HPV vaccine is a safe and effective way to protect against HPV-related cancers. The vaccine is given in a series of two or three shots, depending on the type of vaccine, and is recommended for individuals ages 9-26. The vaccine works by stimulating the body's immune system to produce an immune response to the HPV virus, which helps protect against future HPV infections. One of the key benefits of HPV vaccination is its ability to prevent cervical cancer. Cervical cancer is a leading cause of cancer deaths among women worldwide, but it is also one of the most preventable types of cancer. The HPV vaccine has been shown to reduce the risk of developing cervical cancer by up to 90%, and it is recommended for all girls and women who have not yet been vaccinated. In addition to protecting against cervical cancer, the HPV vaccine can also prevent other types of HPV-related cancers. For example, the vaccine has been shown to reduce the risk of anal and vaginal cancers in women and the risk of penile and oropharyngeal cancers in men. This makes the HPV vaccine a critical tool in reducing the overall burden of HPV-related cancers. The HPV vaccine is also important for reducing the spread of HPV infections. By reducing the number of individuals who become infected with HPV, the vaccine can help break the chain of transmission and reduce the overall prevalence of HPV infections. This not only protects individuals who are vaccinated, but also those who have not yet been vaccinated, as well as those who are unable to receive the vaccine due to age or other health factors. The HPV vaccine is highly effective, but like all vaccines, it is not 100% effective. This means that it is still possible to develop an HPV-related cancer after receiving the vaccine. However, even if an individual does develop an HPV-related cancer, the vaccine can reduce the severity of the disease and increase the chances of successful treatment. In addition to protecting against HPV-related cancers, the HPV vaccine also has other benefits. For example, the vaccine can reduce the need for invasive cervical cancer screening tests, such as Pap tests, and can reduce the number of abnormal Pap test results and biopsies. This can help reduce the emotional and physical burden associated with cervical cancer screening. In conclusion, HPV vaccination is an important tool for preventing HPV-related cancers and reducing the spread of HPV infections. The vaccine is safe, effective, and recommended for individuals ages 9-26. By protecting against HPV-related cancers and reducing the need for invasive cervical cancer screening tests, the HPV vaccine can help reduce the overall burden of HPV-related diseases and improve health outcomes for individuals and communities.

RECOGNIZING POTENTIAL CANCER SYMPTOMS AND SEEKING MEDICAL ATTENTION

Recognizing potential cancer symptoms and seeking medical attention is a crucial step in the early detection and treatment of cancer. Cancer is a complex disease that can manifest in various ways, and early detection is often key to improving the chances of successful treatment and survival. Some of the common symptoms of cancer include:

1. Fatigue: Feeling tired or weak can be a symptom of many different types of cancer, including leukemia and lymphoma. This is because cancer cells can use up a lot of energy, leaving the body feeling tired and weak.
2. Pain: Persistent pain that does not go away or is not relieved by over-the-counter pain relievers can be a sign of cancer. This can include bone pain, abdominal pain, and chest pain.
3. Lumps or masses: Feeling a lump or mass in the body can be a sign of cancer. This can include breast lumps, testicular lumps, and neck or throat lumps.
4. Changes in skin or nails: Changes in the skin or nails can also be a sign of cancer. This can include yellowing of the skin or eyes, darkening of the skin, and changes in the appearance of moles or freckles.

5. Unexpected weight loss: Unexpected weight loss is a common symptom of cancer, especially cancers of the digestive system. This can also include loss of appetite and unexplained changes in body weight.

6. Persistent coughing or hoarseness: A persistent cough or hoarseness can be a sign of lung cancer or throat cancer. This can also include changes in the voice or difficulty swallowing.

7. Changes in bowel or bladder habits: Changes in bowel or bladder habits can be a sign of colon, bladder, or prostate cancer. This can include changes in the frequency, urgency, or appearance of stools or urine.

8. Changes in menstrual cycles: Changes in menstrual cycles can be a sign of gynecological cancers, such as cervical or endometrial cancer. This can include irregular periods, heavy bleeding, or spotting.

9. Headaches: Persistent or worsening headaches can be a sign of brain cancer. This can also include changes in vision, speech, or coordination.

10. Persistent fever or infections: Persistent fever or infections can be a sign of cancer, especially cancers of the blood or immune system.

It is important to remember that these symptoms can also be caused by other health conditions, and not all symptoms are the same for every individual. If you experience any of these symptoms, it is important to seek medical attention as soon as possible. Your doctor can perform a thorough evaluation and recommend any necessary tests or treatments. Early detection and treatment of cancer can significantly improve the chances of successful treatment and survival. This is why it is important to be aware of potential cancer symptoms and to seek medical attention as soon as possible if you experience any of these symptoms.

Regular cancer screenings and early detection tests, such as mammograms, Pap tests, and colon cancer screenings, can also help increase the chances of early detection and successful treatment. Recognizing potential cancer symptoms and seeking medical attention is a critical step in the early detection and treatment of cancer. By being aware of the common symptoms of cancer, individuals can take control of their health and improve their chances of successful treatment and survival. Regular cancer screenings and early detection tests, along with seeking medical attention if you experience any potential cancer symptoms, can help increase the chances of early detection and successful treatment of cancer.

BENEFITS OF CANCER PREVENTION AND EARLY DETECTION FOR OVERALL HEALTH OUTCOMES

Cancer prevention and early detection are crucial for overall health outcomes. By taking proactive measures to reduce the risk of developing cancer and detecting cancer in its early stages, individuals can greatly improve their chances of successful treatment and recovery.

1. Improved Survival Rates: Early detection of cancer increases the chances of successful treatment and survival. When cancer is detected in its early stages, it is often easier to treat and the chances of a successful outcome are higher.

2. Reduced Treatment Costs: Early detection of cancer can reduce treatment costs by reducing the need for more aggressive and expensive treatments, such as surgery and chemotherapy. Early detection can also reduce the need for long-term care, such as hospitalization and rehabilitation, which can be expensive.

3. Better Quality of Life: Early detection and treatment of cancer can improve the quality of life for individuals and their families. By detecting cancer in its early stages, individuals can avoid the discomfort and distress associated with more advanced stages of cancer, and can also

minimize the impact of cancer on their daily lives and activities.

4. Lower Mortality Rates: Cancer prevention and early detection can help lower mortality rates. By reducing the risk of developing cancer and detecting it in its early stages, individuals can reduce their chances of dying from cancer.

5. Improved Health Outcomes: Cancer prevention and early detection can improve overall health outcomes. By reducing the risk of developing cancer and detecting it early, individuals can reduce their chances of developing other health problems, such as heart disease and stroke, which are often associated with cancer.

6. Increased Awareness: Cancer prevention and early detection can increase awareness about the importance of taking control of one's health. By learning about the risk factors for cancer and the benefits of early detection, individuals can become more knowledgeable about their health and more proactive in seeking care and treatment.

7. Better Emotional Well-being: Cancer prevention and early detection can improve emotional well-being by reducing the fear and anxiety associated with a cancer diagnosis. By knowing that they are taking proactive measures to reduce their risk of developing cancer and detect it early, individuals can feel more confident and in control of their health.

8. Improved Family Relationships: Cancer prevention and early detection can improve family relationships by reducing the stress and burden associated with caring for a loved one with cancer. By detecting cancer early, families can better support their loved one and help them manage their health and treatment.

Cancer prevention and early detection offer numerous benefits for overall health outcomes. By reducing the risk of developing cancer and detecting it early, individuals can improve their chances of successful treatment and recovery, reduce treatment costs, improve their quality of life, lower mortality rates, improve overall health outcomes, increase awareness, improve emotional well-being, and improve family relationships. By taking proactive measures to prevent cancer and detect it early, individuals can take control of their health and improve their chances of a successful outcome.

Importance of maintaining a healthy body weight

Maintaining a healthy body weight is crucial for overall health and well-being. By keeping a healthy weight, individuals can reduce their risk of developing numerous health problems, including cancer, heart disease, stroke, and diabetes.

1. Reduced Risk of Chronic Diseases: Maintaining a healthy body weight can help reduce the risk of chronic diseases, such as cancer, heart disease, stroke, and diabetes. By keeping a healthy weight, individuals can reduce their chances of developing these diseases and improve their chances of a long, healthy life.

2. Improved Physical Health: Maintaining a healthy body weight can improve physical health by reducing the risk of injury and promoting physical activity. By keeping a healthy weight, individuals can reduce the risk of developing health problems, such as joint pain and back pain, and can also improve their physical function and mobility.

3. Improved Mental Health: Maintaining a healthy body weight can also improve mental health. By keeping a healthy weight, individuals can reduce the risk of developing mental health problems, such as anxiety and

depression, and can also improve their mood and self-esteem.

4. Better Quality of Life: Maintaining a healthy body weight can improve the quality of life by reducing the risk of health problems and promoting physical and mental well-being. By keeping a healthy weight, individuals can enjoy a better quality of life and can participate in activities that they enjoy.

5. Increased Longevity: Maintaining a healthy body weight can increase longevity. By reducing the risk of developing health problems and promoting physical and mental well-being, individuals can live longer, healthier life.

6. Improved Energy Levels: Maintaining a healthy body weight can also improve energy levels. By keeping a healthy weight, individuals can reduce the risk of fatigue and increase their energy levels, allowing them to be more active and productive.

7. Reduced Medical Costs: Maintaining a healthy body weight can also reduce medical costs. By reducing the risk of developing health problems, individuals can reduce the need for medical care and treatment, and can also avoid the financial burden of medical expenses.

8. Better Sleep: Maintaining a healthy body weight can also improve sleep. By reducing the risk of developing health problems, individuals can improve their sleep quality and avoid sleep disturbances, allowing them to feel more refreshed and energized.

In conclusion, maintaining a healthy body weight is crucial for overall health and well-being. By reducing the risk of chronic diseases, improving physical and mental health, improving the quality of life, increasing longevity, improving energy levels, reducing medical costs, and improving sleep, individuals can greatly improve their chances of a long, healthy life. By making healthy lifestyle choices, such as eating a balanced diet and participating in physical activity, individuals can take control of their health and maintain a healthy weight.

Limiting exposure to known carcinogens (e.g. air pollution, chemicals)

Limiting exposure to known carcinogens is a critical aspect of cancer prevention. Carcinogens are substances or agents that are capable of causing cancer. Exposure to these substances can increase the risk of developing cancer.

1. Air Pollution: Air pollution is a known carcinogen that is widely prevalent in many urban areas. Exposure to air pollution can increase the risk of lung cancer, as well as other respiratory and cardiovascular diseases. To limit exposure to air pollution, individuals should avoid spending time in heavily polluted areas, such as near highways, and should use air purifiers in their homes.

2. Chemicals: Exposure to certain chemicals can also increase the risk of cancer. For example, exposure to certain pesticides and herbicides, as well as industrial chemicals, such as benzene and asbestos, can increase the risk of developing cancer. To limit exposure to these chemicals, individuals should be aware of the chemicals that are commonly used in their work or home environment and should take steps to limit their exposure.

3. Tobacco: Tobacco smoke contains numerous carcinogens, including tar, carbon monoxide, and heavy metals. Exposure to tobacco smoke can increase the risk of developing lung cancer, as well as other respiratory and cardiovascular diseases. To limit exposure to tobacco smoke, individuals should avoid smoking and should avoid being in areas where tobacco smoke is present.

4. Radiation: Exposure to radiation, such as ultraviolet (UV) radiation from the sun, can also increase the risk of cancer. To limit radiation exposure, individuals should protect their skin from the sun by wearing protective clothing and using sunblock, and should also limit their exposure to X-rays and other sources of radiation.

5. Food Contaminants: Certain food contaminants, such as mycotoxins, acrylamides, and phthalates, can also increase the risk of cancer. To limit exposure to these contaminants, individuals should consume a balanced diet that is rich in fruits, vegetables, and whole grains, and should also avoid consuming processed foods that contain preservatives and other chemicals.

6. Water Contaminants: Exposure to certain water contaminants, such as heavy metals, can also increase the risk of cancer. To limit exposure to these contaminants, individuals should use a water filtration system and should also be aware of the water sources that are most likely to contain contaminants.

In conclusion, limiting exposure to known carcinogens is a critical aspect of cancer prevention. By being aware of the substances and agents that can increase the risk of cancer, individuals can take steps to limit their exposure and reduce their risk of developing cancer. By making healthy lifestyle choices, such as eating a balanced diet, participating in physical activity, and avoiding exposure to tobacco smoke and other known carcinogens, individuals can reduce their risk of developing cancer and improve their chances of a long, healthy life.

23

ABOUT THE AUTHOR

Diane T. Norwood is a talented and dedicated writer, known for her passion for the written word and her commitment to crafting well-researched, insightful pieces. With a unique perspective and a talent for bringing complex ideas to life. Whether writing about current events, personal experiences, or social issues, Diane brings a wealth of knowledge and a distinct voice to every project. Her passion for writing and her commitment to excellence has made him a sought-after writer, and her work continues to inspire and inform readers everywhere.

www.ingramcontent.com/pod-product-compliance
Lightning Source LLC
Chambersburg PA
CBHW061559250726
48657CB00021B/2408